The Longevity Road Map

Techniques for Living a Happy and Healthful Life

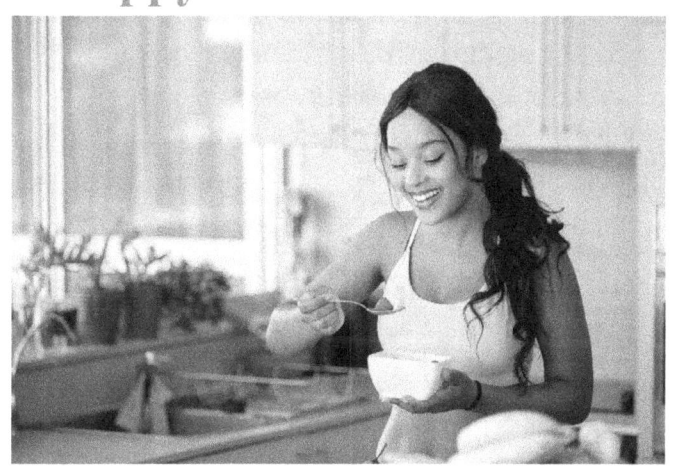

By

Sarah Evans

Table of contents

Introduction

The pursuit of longevity has evolved into more than just a desire in a world where the pace of life appears to be increasing on a daily basis; it's a mission for a more extravagant, better presence. Welcome to "The Longevity road map " - a thorough aid that rises above customary wellbeing stories, offering you a guide to living longer as well as living better.

Meaning of Longevity:

Life span, at its center, alludes to the term of an individual's life. In any case, with regards to our excursion, it reaches out past simple endurance. It typifies personal satisfaction, incorporating actual essentialness, smartness, and profound prosperity. Life span isn't just about the amount of years yet the wealth of encounters and the capacity to relish each experience with zeal.

Significance of Life span in Health:

Why should our pursuit of well-being prioritize longevity? The response lies in the unpredictable association between a more extended life and a better life. Dragging out our years isn't an objective in seclusion; it is interlaced with the goal for a daily existence set apart by essentialness, versatility, and satisfaction.

As we dig into the subtleties of life span, we unwind the significant effect it can have on our wellbeing. Stretched out years present a potential chance to participate in additional significant connections, seek after interests, and add to the world.

Besides, a more drawn out life gives the material to carry out better way of life decisions, lessening the gamble of constant sicknesses and improving in general prosperity.

Outline of the Lifespan Street Map:

"The Longevity road map" isn't simply a book; it's your believed sidekick on the excursion to a better, seriously satisfying life. The road map that can be found on these pages is an all-encompassing strategy that addresses the physical, mental, emotional, and even environmental aspects of well-being.

This guide is definitely not a one-size-fits-all arrangement. It perceives the uniqueness of every person and guides you in making a customized plan custom-made to your necessities. It's not about making radical changes; rather, it's about making changes that last and become part of your daily routine, bringing you long-term benefits.

As we set out on this excursion together, expect to uncover the mysteries of mitigating calories, tackling the force of superfoods, investigating animating work-out schedules, and diving into pressure the board strategies.

" The Life span Guide" is in excess of an aid; it's an encouragement to change your way to deal with wellbeing and embrace an existence of enduring essentialness.

Come along with us as we navigate the complex web of lifestyle choices, environmental influences, and genetics. Figure out how to interpret the code of life span inserted inside your DNA and find the possibility to broaden your life expectancy as well as your healthspan.

This book is in excess of a manual; it's a discussion about the significant crossing point of science and common sense. It's tied in with assuming responsibility for your prosperity and understanding that every choice you make affects the length and nature of your life.

We will learn about the nutritional strategies that can help you on your journey, the significance of good sleep and physical health, and the secrets to mental and emotional well-being in the chapters that come after. We will wander into preventive medical services measures, investigate the effect of ecological variables on life span, and examine the job of innovation in improving our prosperity.

"The Longevity road map" isn't simply a manual for a more extended life; it's an engaging instrument that furnishes you with the information to settle on informed decisions, embrace extraordinary ways of life, and set out on an excursion toward a better, more energetic you.

Thus, we should turn the page together and start this extraordinary undertaking. The way to lifespan is before us, and the conceivable outcomes are limitless. Might it be said that you are prepared to reclassify how you might interpret wellbeing and embrace a day to day existence set apart by getting through essentialness? The experience is standing by.

Section one: Groundworks of Life span

A. Hereditary qualities and Maturing

In the mind boggling dance of life, our hereditary code holds the way to numerous secrets, including the maturing system. Understanding the exchange among hereditary qualities and life span is principal as we leave on our mission for a better, seriously persevering through life.

Unraveling the Hereditary Blueprint:
Hereditary qualities shape our inclination to specific ailments, affecting how our bodies age. " The Longevity road map" dives into the interesting universe of genomics, unwinding the many-sided strands that add to the maturing system.

By understanding our hereditary cosmetics, we gain experiences into potential well being dangers and open doors for proactive intercessions.

Epigenetics and Way of life Influence:
While our qualities give the underlying content, way of life decisions and ecological elements can alter the story. Epigenetics, the investigation of

changes in quality articulation, uncovers how our ways of behaving and climate can impact the maturing direction. The empowering idea that our choices can alter genetic outcomes, paving the way for a longer and healthier life, is the focus of this chapter.

Techniques for Hereditary Wellness:
"The Longevity road map" gives noteworthy systems to upgrade hereditary wellbeing. From customized sustenance designs that line up with hereditary profiles to way of life adjustments that supplement hereditary qualities, this segment furnishes you with the devices to saddle the force of your qualities in advancing life span.

B. Natural Variables

Our general surroundings apply a significant effect on our prosperity, impacting how we age and the nature of our lives. Understanding and moderating ecological variables is an essential step in our life span venture.

Air and Water Quality:
In a period set apart by industrialization, the air we inhale and the water we drink assume significant parts in our wellbeing. This part investigates the significance of clean air and water, offering useful

hints to limit openness to contaminations and poisons. Figure out how little changes in your current circumstance can add to a huge improvement in your general prosperity.

Living Spaces and Longevity:
Our prompt environmental elements, from the home to the work environment, essentially influence our wellbeing. " The Longevity road map" guides you through making living spaces helpful for prosperity, accentuating the job of normal light, vegetation, and cleaned up spaces in advancing life span.

Reasonable Practices:
Natural maintainability is interlaced with individual life span. This section examines eco-accommodating practices that add to a better planet as well as encourage a better you. Find how maintainable living decisions can decidedly impact your prosperity and add to the more extensive objective of life span.

C. Way of life Decisions

Our day to day choices go about as a compass, directing us toward either a way of wellbeing or one of potential wellbeing challenges. " The Longevity Road Map" complicatedly analyzes way of life decisions, offering experiences into what little changes can prompt huge means for one's life span.

Nourishment as a Foundation:
Investigate the transformative effects of nutrition on longevity. This segment not just separates the advantages of calming slims down yet in addition gives useful hints to integrating life span improving superfoods into your dinners. Reveal the job of discontinuous fasting and caloric limitation in improving your body's normal cycles for supported wellbeing.

Exercise for a Long Life:
Actual work is a foundation of life span. Whether you're a wellness lover or a beginner, "The Longevity road map" gives custom fitted activity proposals, underlining the significance of both cardiovascular and strength-preparing works out. Figure out how a fair way to deal with wellness can sustain your body against the impacts of maturing.

Stress The executives Techniques:
If stress is not controlled, it can be a silent enemy of longevity. This segment demonstrates the pressure of the executives' methods, from care practices to unwinding works out, furnishing you with the instruments to explore life's difficulties while keeping up with your prosperity.

In section one, we establish the groundwork for your life span venture by analyzing the mind boggling balance between hereditary qualities, climate, and way of life.

Not only is "The Longevity Road Map" a book, it's a manual for opening the mysteries of a more extended, better life.

As we explore these fundamental viewpoints, expect reasonable bits of knowledge, engaging procedures, and a reestablished viewpoint on the boundless opportunities for your wellbeing and life span. The excursion has recently started, and the street ahead is loaded up with disclosure. Might it be said that you are prepared to make the following stride?

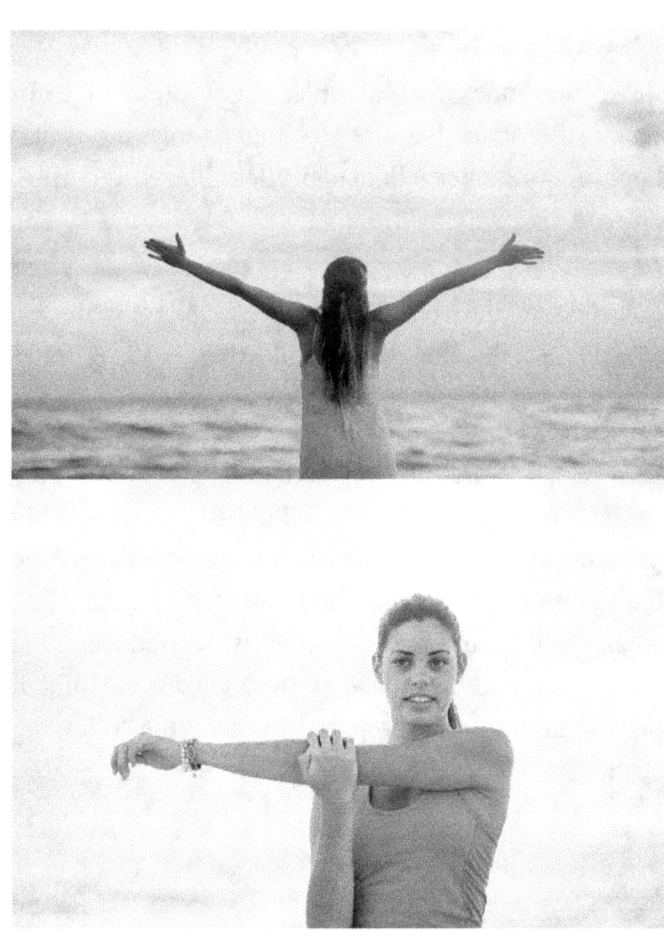

Section Two: Nutritional Methods

A. Anti-Inflammatory Diets

Unlocking the secrets of longevity begins at the table, where our choices can either fuel inflammation or promote a healthy body balance. In this part, we dive into the extraordinary force of calming counts calories as a foundation for improving your health span.

Grasping Inflammation:
Numerous age-related diseases are increasingly being linked to chronic inflammation. The Life span Guide" reveals insight into the instruments of aggravation, representing how dietary decisions can either worsen or ease this interior pressure.

Learn more about the connection between conditions like heart disease, arthritis, and cognitive decline and inflammation.

Anti-inflammatory diet components:
Investigate a different exhibit of food varieties that structure the groundwork of calming slims down. From omega-3 unsaturated fats found in greasy fish

to the cell reinforcement rich properties of leafy foods, this part gives a far reaching manual for building dinners that control irritation and backing your body's regular recuperating processes.

Useful Hints for Implementation:
Progressing to a mitigating diet doesn't need to overpower. " The Longevity road map" offers pragmatic tips and feast plans to flawlessly coordinate these healthful systems into your regular routine. Find how little, supportable changes can prompt critical upgrades in your general prosperity.

B. Superfoods for Life span

Nature has given us an abundance of supplement thick superfoods, each offering an extraordinary arrangement of medical advantages. In this part, we reveal the superheroes of nourishment - food varieties that go past simple food to add to a more drawn out, better life.

Investigating Superfoods:
From energetic berries plentiful in cell reinforcements to mixed greens overflowing with nutrients and minerals, "The Longevity road map" acquaints you with a range of superfoods. Each superfood is a dietary force to be reckoned with, assuming a fundamental part in bracing your body

against the impacts of maturing and advancing ideal wellbeing.

Recipes and Culinary Adventures:
Hoist your culinary involvement in flavorful and supporting recipes consolidating these superfoods. Whether you're a carefully prepared culinary expert or a kitchen beginner, this part gives motivation and direction on getting ready dinners that entice your taste buds as well as add to your life span venture.

Coordinating Superfoods into Your Diet:
Reasonableness is at the core of "The Longevity road map." Figure out how to flawlessly coordinate superfoods into your day to day feasts, guaranteeing that your nourishing decisions line up with your objective of a more extended, better life. You will be able to plan your meals and navigate grocery store aisles with confidence thanks to this chapter.

C. Irregular Fasting and Caloric Limitation

Past the substance of our plates, the timing and amount of our feasts can essentially influence life span. This part investigates the ideas of irregular fasting and caloric limitation - nourishing techniques that stretch out past what you eat to when and the amount you eat.

Fasting intermittently:

Reveal the science behind discontinuous fasting, a training that substitutes times of eating with times of fasting. " The Longevity road map" gives bits of knowledge into what irregular fasting means for metabolic wellbeing, advances cell fix, and adds to life span. Investigate various ways to deal with irregular fasting, permitting you to find a strategy that lines up with your way of life.

Limitations on Calories and Longevity:

Plunge into the interesting domain of caloric limitation, a dietary methodology that includes diminishing calorie consumption without compromising fundamental supplements. Comprehend the components by which caloric limitation might slow the maturing system, upgrade cell flexibility, and possibly expand your healthspan. Viable ways to carry out caloric limitation in a practical way are likewise given.

Adjusting Nourishing Strategies:

Balance is emphasized in "The Longevity Road Map." Find how calming eats less, superfoods, discontinuous fasting, and caloric limitation can synergistically cooperate to make a healthful starting point for life span. This part directs you in making a customized approach that thinks about your one of a kind inclinations, wellbeing objectives, and way of life.

In Section Two, we explore the multifaceted scene of dietary systems, where each nibble is a potential chance to fuel your excursion toward a more drawn out, better life. " The Longevity Road Map" engages you to settle on careful decisions, guaranteeing that your healthful establishment isn't simply supporting life however improving it.

As you leave this section, expect a culinary experience injected with science, common sense, and the commitment of extraordinary prosperity. Is it safe to say that you are prepared to relish the kinds of life span?

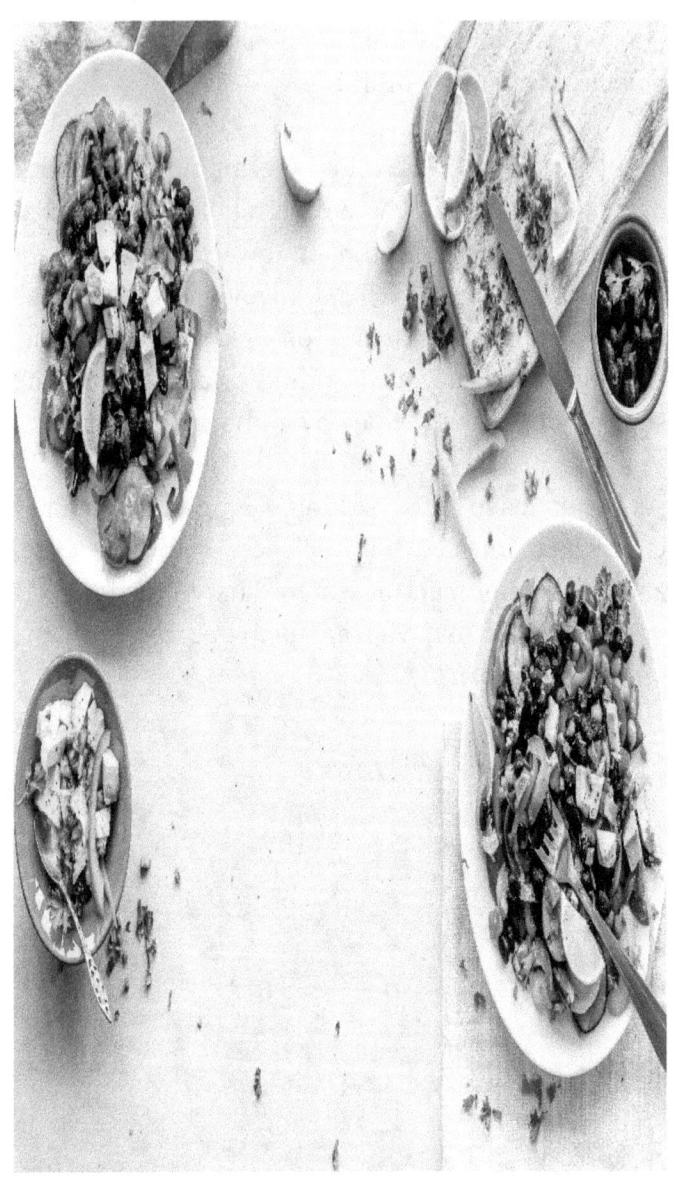

Section Three: Actual Health

A. Exercise and Lifespan

Leaving on the way to lifespan includes something beyond dietary decisions; it requires a functioning obligation to actual health. In this section, "The Longevity road map" investigates the cooperative connection among practice and a more extended, better life.

Understanding the Benefits of Physical Activity:
Practice isn't simply a way to keep an alluring build; it is an integral asset in advancing generally speaking prosperity. Learn how the science behind regular physical activity improves cardiovascular health, increases mental acuity, and even slows down cellular aging.

Adjusting Cardiovascular and Strength Training:
"The Longevity road map" advocates for a comprehensive way to deal with work out, incorporating both cardiovascular and strength-preparing exercises.

Find the advantages of cardio exercises in keeping up with heart wellbeing and investigate strength preparing as a way to safeguard bulk, bone thickness, and metabolic capability - vital components in the life span condition.

Adapting exercise to individual requirements:
This section offers advice on adapting exercise routines to individual preferences, abilities, and health conditions in light of the fact that every person is different. "The Longevity Road Map" gives you the tools to create a long-term exercise plan that fits your lifestyle, whether you're an avid fitness enthusiast or just starting out.

B. Significance of Rest

In the rushing about of present day life, rest frequently assumes a lower priority. However, the quality and term of our rest assume a crucial part in deciding the direction of our wellbeing and life span. This segment enlightens the meaning of focusing on rest as a foundation of actual wellbeing.

Unloading the Rest Life span Connection:
Investigate the intricate connection between longevity and sleep. The Life span Guide" demystifies the science behind how satisfactory, serene rest adds to cell fix, chemical guideline, and

mental capability. Learn how sleep affects immune health and how it helps prevent chronic diseases.

Improving Rest Hygiene:
Establishing a climate helpful for quality rest is a fundamental part of actual wellbeing. This part gives viable tips to enhancing your rest cleanliness - from making a quieting sleep time routine to laying out a rest cordial room. Find out how these adjustments can make your sleep deeper and more restorative.

Addressing Sleep Problems and Obstacles:
For those wrestling with rest problems or confronting difficulties in accomplishing peaceful rest, "The Longevity road map" offers experiences into distinguishing and resolving these issues. From rest apnea to sleep deprivation, this part gives direction on looking for proficient assistance and carrying out way of life changes to further develop rest quality.

C. Stress The board Strategies

Stress, whenever left unrestrained, can turn into a quiet saboteur of life span. Perceiving its effect on physical and mental prosperity, "The Longevity road map" devotes a part to pressure the executives methods - enabling you to explore life's difficulties with strength.

Grasping the Pressure Lifespan Connection:
Numerous health issues, including cardiovascular problems and impaired immune function, are linked to chronic stress. This section investigates the physiological and mental impacts of weight on the body and underlines the significance of taking on proactive measures to pressure the executives.

Care Practices for Pressure Reduction:
In "The Longevity Road Map," mindfulness is presented as an effective method for reducing stress. From contemplation and profound breathing activities to careful development rehearses like yoga, find how integrating these strategies into your routine can cultivate close to home equilibrium and strengthen your psychological prosperity.

Relaxation from Stress Through Physical Activity:
In addition to being an essential component of physical health, exercise is a natural stress reliever.

Figure out how participating in normal actual work assists with lightening pressure, decrease nervousness, and improve your general state of mind. " The Life span Guide" gives viable tips to incorporating exercise into your daily schedule to stress the executives.

In Section Three, we shift our concentration to the domain of actual health, perceiving that a flourishing body is crucial to a flourishing life.

" The Longevity Road Map" guides you through the interconnected components of activity, rest, and stress of the executives, offering useful bits of knowledge and customized methodologies to upgrade your actual prosperity.

 As you explore this part, imagine a daily existence where your body endures the progression of time as well as twists with essentialness. Might it be said that you are prepared to embrace actual health as a foundation of your life span venture?

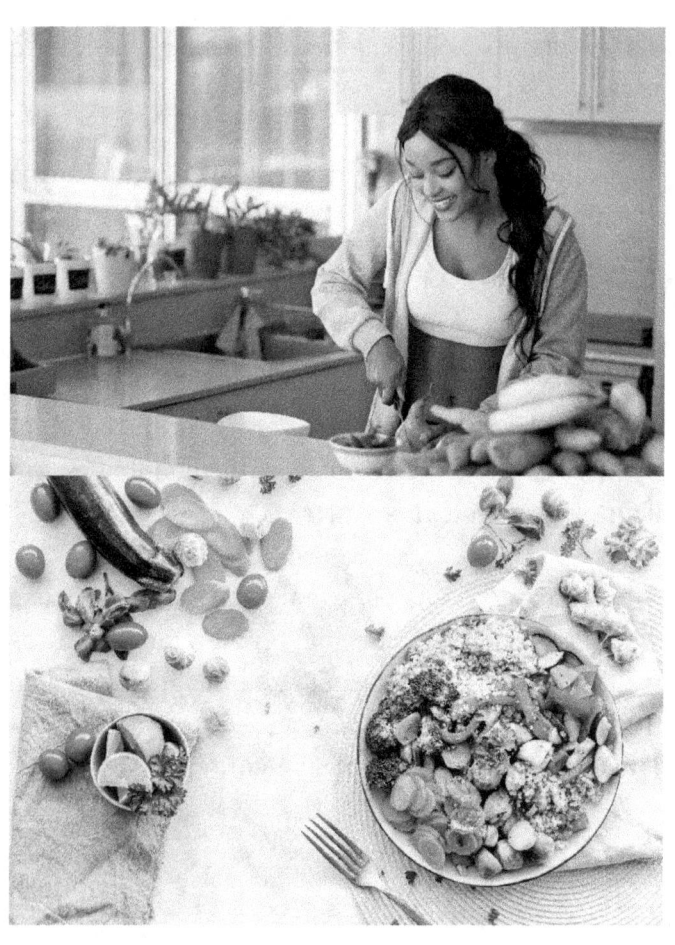

Section Four: Mental and Close to home Prosperity

A. Mental Wellbeing Tips

In the complex embroidery of life span, smartness and mental wellbeing are strings that wind through the texture of a satisfying life. The fourth chapter of "The Longevity Road Map" looks at cognitive health tips that can help you keep and improve your mental faculties.

Sustaining Your Brain:
The mind, a wonder of intricacy, requires legitimate sustenance for supported capability. " The Longevity road map" unfurls mental wellbeing tips that envelop a scope of way of life decisions, from nourishment techniques that help cerebrum wellbeing to participating in mental activities that invigorate mental capability.

Practice for the Mind:
Similarly as actual activity reinforces the body, mental activities sustain the brain. This part presents various mental exercises - from riddles and games to acquiring new abilities - intended to keep your

mind coordinated and versatile. Find how taking on an inquisitive outlook can add to mental life span.

Quality Rest and Mental Function:
The significance of rest reaches out past actual prosperity; it is a foundation of mental wellbeing. Figure out how adequate and relaxing rest upholds memory union, critical thinking abilities, and generally speaking mental lucidity. " The Longevity Road Map" offers experiences enhancing rest for mental advantages.

B. Profound Flexibility

Embracing life span isn't just about actual wellbeing; likewise developing profound strength permits you to explore life's difficulties with beauty and guts. This part of the section digs into techniques for upgrading profound prosperity.

Understanding Close to home Resilience:
Close to home flexibility is the capacity to return from affliction and keep up with mental prosperity despite life's highs and lows. " The Longevity Road Map" investigates the parts of profound flexibility, revealing insight into the attitude and practices that add to close to home strength.

Mind-Body Connection:

The brain and body are complicatedly associated, and feelings can influence actual wellbeing. This segment gives experiences into the psyche body association, underlining practices, for example, care and contemplation that advance close to home equilibrium. Find how developing a positive close to home state adds to general prosperity.

Down to earth Devices for Profound Resilience:
"The Longevity road map" furnishes you with commonsense apparatuses for developing close to home strength.

From journaling and appreciation practices to cultivating a positive social climate, investigate significant methodologies that enable you to explore stressors and misfortunes while keeping up with close to home harmony.

C. Social Associations and Life span

People are innately friendly animals, and the nature of our social associations assumes a critical part in forming our general prosperity. Part 4 finishes up with an emphasis on the effect of social associations on life span.

The Social-Life span Link:

Research reliably shows areas of strength that associations are related with expanded life span. " The Longevity Road Map focuses on the significance of meaningful relationships in the pursuit of a longer and healthier life by examining the mechanisms by which social interactions influence physical and mental health.

Assembling and Sustaining Relationships:
This part gives direction on building and supporting social associations that go past superficial connections. From encouraging dear companionships to keeping up with family ties, "The Longevity road map" offers down to earth tips on making a strong interpersonal organization that adds to your general prosperity.

Participation of the Community and Goal:
Past individual connections, commitment with more extensive networks and a feeling of direction contribute essentially to life span.

 Investigate how contribution in local area exercises, humanitarian effort, or chasing after significant objectives can upgrade your psychological and profound prosperity, eventually advancing a feeling of satisfaction and life span.

In Section Four, we jump profound into the domains of mental and close to home prosperity, perceiving the significant effect these viewpoints have on the excursion toward a more extended, better life. " The Longevity road map" welcomes you to focus on mental wellbeing, develop close to home flexibility, and support significant social associations.

As you explore this part, imagine a day to day existence rich with mental lucidity, profound strength, and strong connections. Is it safe to say that you are prepared to embrace the keys to mental and profound life span?

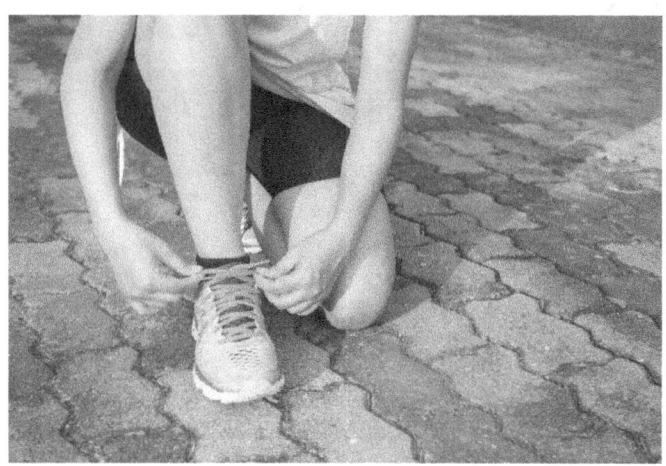

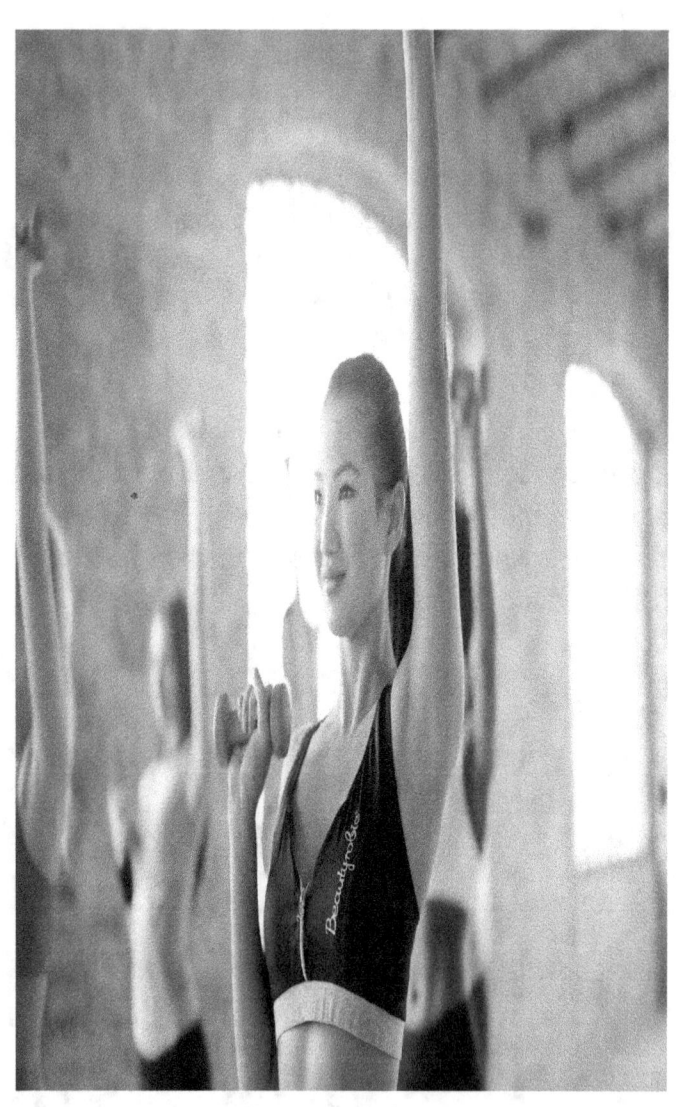

Section Five: Preventive Medical services

Chasing after life span, proactive and preventive medical care measures arise as significant components in safeguarding prosperity and preparing for potential wellbeing challenges. Section five of "The Longevity Road Map" is devoted to investigating the meaning of preventive medical care, covering standard check-ups, immunizations, and the administration of persistent circumstances.

A. Customary Check-ups and Screenings

The Groundwork of Prevention:
Preventive medical care starts with mindfulness and ordinary checking of your wellbeing. " The Longevity Road Map stresses how important it is to schedule regular checkups to catch problems early.

Standard wellbeing evaluations act as a proactive way to deal with keeping up with ideal prosperity, considering convenient mediations and way of life changes.

Early Detection Screenings:

This part directs you through different wellbeing screenings that are instrumental in identifying potential medical problems before side effects emerge.

From pulse checks and cholesterol screenings to disease screenings and diabetes evaluations, "The Longevity road map" gives a far reaching outline of screenings that can fundamentally influence your preventive medical care system.

Plans for individual prevention:
Understanding that every individual is one of a kind, this part underlines the significance of customized counteraction plans. " The Longevity road map" investigates how fitting preventive techniques in light of individual wellbeing profiles and chance variables upgrades the viability of early location and mediation.

B. Inoculations and Vaccinations

The Force of Vaccination:
Immunizations are not only a youth need; they assume a crucial part in preventive medical care over the course of life. The significance of vaccinations in preventing infectious diseases is discussed in depth in this section. The Longevity road map" frames suggested inoculations for

various age gatherings and investigates how keeping awake to-date with vaccinations adds to generally speaking wellbeing and life span.

Resistant Wellbeing and Longevity:
Understanding the association between a powerful safe framework and life span is fundamental.

" The Longevity road map" gives bits of knowledge into how immunizations reinforce the invulnerable reaction, lessening the gamble of extreme ailment and inconveniences. The broader effects of immune health on overall health are examined in this section.

Exploring Discussions and Concerns:
Vaccinations can occasionally provoke debate and concern. This part tends to normal confusions, giving proof based data to enable informed independent direction. " The Longevity road map" stresses the job of immunizations in individual wellbeing as well as in adding to group resistance and local area prosperity.

C.   Overseeing   Ongoing Circumstances

Ongoing Circumstances and Longevity:

Constant circumstances, like diabetes, hypertension, and coronary illness, can essentially affect both the quality and length of life. " The Longevity road map" recognizes the predominance of ongoing circumstances and underscores the significance of compelling administration chasing life span.

This part investigates how early conclusion, way of life adjustments, and clinical mediations can moderate the effect of persistent sicknesses.

All encompassing Way to deal with Management:
Adopting a comprehensive strategy to ongoing conditions on the board is vital. This chapter examines how to manage chronic conditions by changing one's lifestyle, such as eating better, exercising, and managing stress.

The Life span Guide" gives functional tips to making a comprehensive administration plan that upgrades by and large prosperity.

The Job of Standard Monitoring:

Reliable observing of constant circumstances is fundamental for compelling administration. " The Longevity Road Map" guides people on the significance of ordinary check-ups, observing key wellbeing markers, and teaming up with medical services experts to change the executives' systems depending on the situation.

This proactive methodology guarantees that ongoing circumstances are very much made due, advancing life span and a top notch of life.

In Chapter Five, "The Longevity Road Map," the significance of preventative healthcare in extending lives is emphasized.

Standard check-ups, inoculations, and the viable administration of constant circumstances are parts of a far reaching wellbeing system as well as demonstrations of taking care of oneself that establish the groundwork for a better and longer life.

 As you explore this part, imagine a proactive way to deal with wellbeing that enables you to assume responsibility for your prosperity. Is it safe to say that you are prepared to embrace preventive medical care as a foundation of your life span venture?

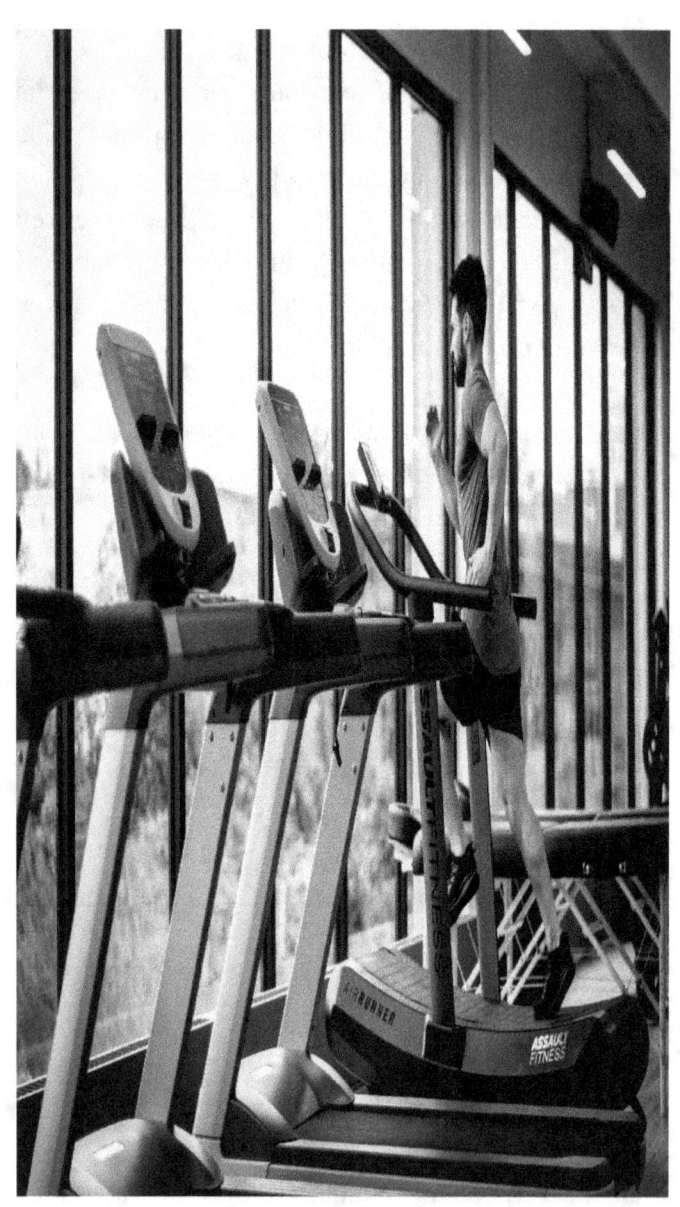

Section Six: Ecological Variables

In this significant part, we dig into the complex exchange between our living climate and our general prosperity.

The climate we occupy altogether influences our wellbeing, both for the time being and throughout the span of our lives. This section investigates three vital elements of natural variables: Sustainable practices for long-term viability, air and water quality, and clean living spaces.

A. Clean Living Spaces

1. The Effect of Messiness on Psychological well-being
- Looking at the mental cost of messiness on mental prosperity.
- Down to earth methodologies for cleaning up and coordinating living spaces for working on mental capability.

2. Indoor Air Quality
- Disentangling the risks of indoor contaminations and their consequences for respiratory wellbeing.
- Making use of plants that purify the air and putting in place efficient ventilation systems.

3. Normal Lighting and its Impact

- Exploring the physiological advantages of openness to regular light.

- Planning living spaces to amplify admittance to regular light for temperament upgrade.

B. Air and Water Quality

1. Outside Air Quality

- Figuring out the effect of open air contamination on wellbeing.

- Promoting environmentally friendly methods of reducing air pollution in local communities.

2. Water Quality and Human Wellbeing

- Dissecting the meaning of clean water for general wellbeing.

- Making people aware of problems with water contamination and arguing for easy access to clean drinking water

3. The Job of Green Spaces

- Investigating the medical advantages of green spaces and nature submersion.

- In urban planning, encouraging the creation and upkeep of parks and other green spaces.

C. Feasible Practices for Life span

1. Supportable Dietary patterns
- Inspecting the natural effect of dietary decisions.
- Empowering plant-based consumes less calories and investigating reasonable food obtaining.

2. Eco-accommodating Living
- Presenting maintainable practices for squander decrease and reusing.
- Featuring the significance of picking harmless to the ecosystem items in day to day existence.

3. The Association Among Ecological and Individual Maintainability
- Underscoring the cooperative connection between private prosperity and ecological manageability.
- Pushing for cognizant way of life decisions that add to both individual life span and the soundness of the planet.

This chapter concludes by emphasizing the significant impact of our environment on our health and longevity. Clean living spaces, perfect air and water quality, and supportable practices are fundamental for our own prosperity as well as imperative for the drawn out strength of our planet. We pave the way for a healthier and more sustainable future for ourselves and future generations by comprehending and implementing these environmental factors.

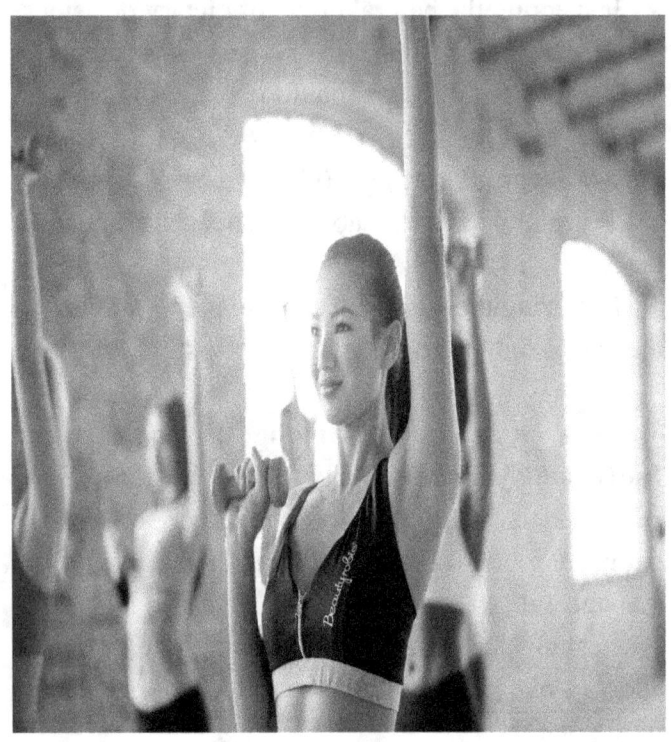

Section seven: Technology and Longevity

In a world where advancements in technology are constantly redefining human capabilities, Chapter Seven delves into the relationship between longevity and technology.

This vital section investigates the job of state of the art developments in forming the scene of medical care, offering a brief look into the encouraging eventual fate of expanded life expectancies.

A. Wearable Wellbeing Tech: Changing Customized Healthcare

The section starts off with a top to bottom examination of wearable wellbeing innovation, an extraordinary power in the mission for life span.

From smartwatches that screen fundamental signs to wellness trackers that flawlessly incorporate into day to day existence, wearables are turning out to be progressively modern. The story moves forward by looking at how these gadgets affect people's ability to manage their health on their own.

The conversation digs into the advancement of wearable wellbeing tech, investigating its foundations in essential movement following its present status of offering constant wellbeing bits of knowledge.

The section exhibits explicit instances of how wearables enable clients to follow their wellness, screen rest designs, and oversee feelings of anxiety. In particular, the narrative places an emphasis on the potential of wearables to identify early warning signs of health issues, encouraging strategies for preventative healthcare.

B. Remote monitoring and telemedicine:

Crossing over Holes in Medical care Access

Pushing ahead, the investigation movements to the domain of telemedicine and remote checking. In a time where the worldwide network is at its apex, these advancements arise as significant apparatuses in guaranteeing medical services availability for all.

The chapter tells the story by looking at how telemedicine broke down geographical barriers and reached populations that were not previously served.

Telemedicine's job in significant distance patient consideration is taken apart, featuring how virtual meetings and remote observing rethink the conventional specialist patient relationship.

Genuine contextual analyses and examples of overcoming adversity represent the viability of telemedicine in constant sickness the board, postoperative consideration, and psychological wellness support.

The chapter emphasizes these technologies' potential to transform healthcare delivery while elucidating the difficulties and ethical considerations associated with them.

C. Innovations in Medical services:

The final section of the chapter, titled "The Longevity road map," takes readers on a journey to the cutting edge of healthcare innovation and highlights developments that have the potential to extend a person's lifespan. From quality altering innovations to man-made intelligence driven diagnostics, the story unfurls the most recent progressions impelling the clinical field into unfamiliar domains.

The part gives an outline of quality treatments and their capability to address hereditary inclinations to infections, offering a brief look into a future where genetic circumstances can be really treated.

Moreover, it investigates the job of man-made reasoning in upsetting diagnostics, drug disclosure, and customized treatment plans. The story adjusts the fervor encompassing these advancements with moral contemplations, welcoming perusers to consider the cultural ramifications of controlling the actual texture of life.

All in all, Section Section fills in as a signal directing pursuers through the synergistic connection among innovation and life span. Telemedicine, wearable health technology, and other ground-breaking innovations in healthcare weave a web that holds the promise of not only extending life but also improving its quality.

As mankind keeps on opening the secrets of wellbeing and maturing, the section flashes consideration on the moral and cultural ramifications of these groundbreaking advancements.

Section Eight: Longevity in Different Cultures

Section Eight delves into the multifaceted relationship between culture and longevity as we navigate the diverse tapestry of human civilization.

This illuminating part investigates the extraordinary practices and viewpoints on maturing across various social orders, revealing insight into the insight implanted in social customs that add to expanded and satisfying lives.

A. Blue Zones and Illustrations Learned:

Divulging the Insider facts of Longevity

The part starts with a charming excursion into the idea of Blue Zones — locales all over the planet where a higher-than-normal number of individuals carry on with remarkably longer lives.

Through fastidious examination and convincing stories, the section disentangles the shared factors that characterize these lifespan areas of interest.

Perusers are drenched in the illustrations gained from Blue Zones, taking apart factors like eating regimen, way of life, and local area elements that add to the surprising life span seen in these districts.

From the plant-based diets of Okinawa to the solid feeling of the local area in Sardinia, each Blue Zone uncovers one kind of knowledge into the craft of improving with age.

The story explores through the science behind these perceptions, stressing the significance of embracing comprehensive way of life changes that resound with the social texture of every local area.

B. Cultural Practices for Life span:

Embracing Respected Wisdom

Expanding on the establishment laid by Blue Zones, the section enlarges its degree to investigate social practices for life span across different social orders. Perusers are acquainted with a kaleidoscope of ceremonies, customs, and way of life decisions that have supported wellbeing and prosperity over ages.

From the tea functions of Japan to the Mediterranean eating regimen of Greece, the account dives into the social subtleties that impact dietary propensities and everyday schedules. It analyzes the job of otherworldliness and care in societies that focus on mental and close to home prosperity as essential parts of life span.

Through spellbinding stories and master experiences, the part underlines the significance of social personality in molding people's viewpoints on maturing and the quest for a satisfying life.

C. Global Points of view on Sound Maturing:

Exploring Difficulties and Opportunities

The last segment of the section expands the focal point to offer an all encompassing perspective on worldwide viewpoints on solid maturing. It examines the assorted difficulties looked by changed societies in the journey for expanded life expectancies, going from financial aberrations to the effect of modernization on customary ways of life.

Perusers are taken on an excursion through differentiating ways to deal with maturing, investigating how social mentalities toward the older impact medical services, social emotionally supportive networks, and intergenerational connections. The part disentangles the intricacies of embracing present day medical care while saving social personalities, underscoring the requirement for socially delicate ways to deal with advanced sound maturing around the world.

All in all, Section Eight fills in as a dazzling investigation of the multifaceted exchange among culture and life span. Blue Zones give substantial instances of how social practices can encourage life span, offering a diagram for people trying to take on better ways of life.

Readers are challenged to reflect on their own cultural contexts and the lessons they can learn from the collective wisdom of humanity as the rich tapestry of global cultural practices depicts the diverse approaches that societies take to aging.

As the mission for life span rises above geological limits, this part welcomes perusers to see the value in the wealth of social variety in molding the human experience of a more drawn out, more significant life.

Section Nine: Monetary Making arrangements for Life span

Chasing a more drawn out and better life, Section Nine dives into the basic part of monetary preparation. As people try to expand their life expectancies, the part fastidiously investigates the monetary contemplations and key monetary choices expected to explore the difficulties and amazing open doors that go with life span.

A. Healthcare Costs in Maturing:

The chapter titled "The Longevity road map" begins with a comprehensive discussion of the rising costs of healthcare as people get older. It enlightens the mind boggling elements of clinical costs as people become older, offering perusers an extensive comprehension of the monetary scene related with life span.

The story separates the different parts of medical services costs, from standard check-ups to particular therapies and prescriptions. It accentuates the significance of expecting potential well being related uses, giving perusers functional bits of knowledge into planning for clinical consideration in the later phases of life. Moreover, the section investigates the effect of developing medical care advances and the job they play in molding future medical services costs.

B. Security in Retirement and Money:

Building an Establishment for the Future

Pushing ahead, the center movements to retirement and monetary security — an essential aspect of making arrangements for life span. The chapter explains the intricacies of retirement planning and the significance of making wise and early financial decisions to ensure a secure and enjoyable future.

The story investigates different retirement reserve funds vehicles, from customary benefits plans to 401(k)s and individual retirement accounts (IRAs). It discusses the significance of diversification and investment strategies that are tailored to each person's risk tolerance and financial objectives.

Furthermore, the part examines the developing idea of retirement, where staged retirements and second professions are turning out to be more common, testing customary thoughts of a proper retirement age.

C. Long-Term Care Arranging:

Expecting and Relieving Future Challenges

The last part of the section addresses the frequently neglected part of long haul care arranging. Perceiving that life span can in some cases bring unanticipated wellbeing challenges, the story gives a thorough investigation of the monetary contemplations related with long haul care.

Perusers are directed through the complexities of long haul care protection, Medicaid, and other monetary apparatuses intended to mitigate the financial weight of expanded medical services needs.

The section underlines the significance of proactive preparation, empowering perusers to think about their inclinations for care, possible living game plans, and the monetary ramifications of different long haul care choices.

Genuine contextual analyses represent the assorted ways people approach long haul care arranging, revealing insight into the decisions and compromises inborn in this basic part of monetary readiness.

In conclusion, Chapter Nine provides individuals navigating the financial terrain of longevity with a crucial compass.

From understanding the subtleties of medical services expenses to creating a versatile retirement plan and tending to the intricacies of long haul care, the section furnishes perusers with the information and prescience expected to pursue informed monetary choices.

As the quest for a more drawn out life becomes interlaced with monetary contemplations, this section gives a guide to accomplishing monetary security, guaranteeing that the later phases of life are described by life span as well as by monetary prosperity and inner harmony.

Section Ten: Assembling Everything

As the peruser sets out on the last part of this groundbreaking excursion, Section Ten fills in as the climax of bits of knowledge and viable methodologies gathered from the first sections. This important section helps people create their individual longevity plan, keep track of their progress, and adjust to the ever-changing health and life landscape.

A. Creating Your Customized Life span Plan:

An Outline for a Satisfying Life

The part unfurls with the fundamental undertaking of making a customized life span plan. Readers are encouraged to think about their own aspirations, values, and circumstances by drawing on the wealth of information presented in earlier chapters.

The story fills in as an aide, helping people in devising an exhaustive game plan that coordinates actual wellbeing, mental prosperity, social associations, and monetary security.

From laying out feasible wellbeing objectives in light of individual inclinations to adjusting monetary systems to long haul targets, the part underscores the all encompassing nature of a life span plan.

Down to earth practices and intuitive components engage users to effectively participate in the arranging system, guaranteeing that the subsequent diagram is an impression of their singular needs.

The story supports that life span isn't just about adding a long time to life however upgrading the nature of those years through deliberate decisions.

B. Tracking Progress:

Exploring the Excursion Toward Longevity

Pushing ahead, the center moves to following advancement — a principal part of any extraordinary undertaking. The chapter provides a road map for staying on course and making informed adjustments by introducing readers to tools and methods for monitoring and evaluating the effectiveness of their longevity plan.

The story investigates the combination of innovation, from wellbeing applications that track actual work to monetary apparatuses that screen venture execution.

It underscores the significance of customary well being check-ups and monetary audits as proactive measures to guarantee that the lifespan plan stays lined up with advancing necessities and objectives.

Genuine examples of overcoming adversity highlight the meaning of steady checking, exhibiting how people can celebrate accomplishments and explore misfortunes on their way toward a more extended, better life.

C. Adapting to Evolving Needs:

Embracing Adaptability in Life span Planning

The last part of the section tends to the certainty of progress and the significance of flexibility chasing after life span. The narrative encourages readers to embrace flexibility as a fundamental principle of their longevity plan by acknowledging that life is dynamic and unpredictable.

Perusers are directed through systems for adjusting to changing wellbeing conditions, advancing monetary scenes, and moving needs. The section investigates the job of versatility in exploring unforeseen difficulties, encouraging a mentality that sees misfortunes as any open doors for development and change.

Through contextual investigations and master bits of knowledge, the story represents how people can proactively adjust their arrangements without neglecting to focus on their overall objectives, guaranteeing that life span stays a dynamic and satisfying excursion.

The culmination of the longevity investigation, Chapter Ten instructs readers on how to put what they have learned into practice. By making a customized life span plan, following advancement, and embracing flexibility, people are enabled to assume responsibility for their excursion toward a more drawn out, better, and more significant life.

As the last pages of the book unfurl, the story urges perusers to see life span not as an objective but rather as a progressing, deliberate pursuit — an excursion improved by their decisions and the flexibility they develop en route.

Conclusion

As we wrap this extraordinary investigation of life span up, the finishing up section fills in as an intelligent space, summing up central issues, offering inspirational statements, and giving a convincing source of inspiration.

The essence of the journey is captured in this final section, empowering readers to adopt the book's guiding principles and practices.

A. Recap of Central issues:

Exploring the Scene of Life span Wisdom

The finishing up part begins with a thorough reiteration of the central issues uncovered in the previous sections.

From the significant experiences acquired from Blue Zones to the many-sided dance among innovation and life span, the story returns to the diverse parts of wellbeing, way of life, money, and culture that add to the quest for a more drawn out and seriously satisfying life.

Perusers are helped to remember the meaning of customized life span plans, accentuating the all encompassing nature of such undertakings. The reiteration discusses the significance of proactive health management, strategic financial planning, and the cultural and societal influences that shape the path toward longer lifespans.

The interconnectedness of these components and their collective impact on the pursuit of longevity are emphasized during this reflective journey.

B. Encouragement for Durable Well Being:

Sustaining the Seeds of Well-being

Expanding on the recap, the story changes into a persuasive talk, offering pursuers uplifting statements as they ponder the conceivable outcomes innate in dependable wellbeing.

The section investigates the mental and close to home elements of embracing a life span outlook, stressing the extraordinary force of positive reasoning and purposeful residing.

Perusers are urged to see life span not as an impossible ideal but rather as an excursion set apart by little, reliable strides towards prosperity. The story dives into the idea of strength, featuring its part in defeating obstructions and mishaps that might emerge on the way to a more extended life.

Through genuine stories and master points of view, the section ingrains a feeling of trust and strengthening, cultivating the conviction that setting out on an excursion towards further developed wellbeing and vitality is rarely past the point of no return.

C. Call to Activity:

Start Your Journey to Longevity Right Now!
The finishing up section crescendos with a reverberating source of inspiration, encouraging perusers to make the principal strides on their life span venture today.

The narrative acts as a catalyst for change, beckoning readers to put the information they've learned in the book to use and set out on an individual exploration of their own potential for a life that lasts longer and is more satisfying.

Reasonable advances and significant exhortation are introduced to direct perusers in starting their life span venture. The chapter gives readers the ability to turn inspiration into concrete, life-enhancing actions, such as initiating financial planning, setting achievable health goals, and adopting cultural practices that align with individual values.

The source of inspiration highlights that life span is certainly not a far off objective however an everyday decision — a promise to sustaining prosperity, developing flexibility, and pursuing deliberate decisions that line up with the craving for a dynamic and broadened life.

In conclusion, this book is a comprehensive guide to navigating the complex terrain of health, culture, finances, and personal development, serving as a compass on the path to longevity.

 As the finishing up section unfurls, perusers are not simply given an end but rather with a greeting — a challenge to set out on a groundbreaking excursion towards a more drawn out, better, and more significant life.

The narrative reinforces the idea that longevity is not a destination to be reached but rather a dynamic and deliberate journey to be embraced—one that begins with a single step and progresses with each conscious choice toward a future that is enhanced by the promise of enduring well-being.

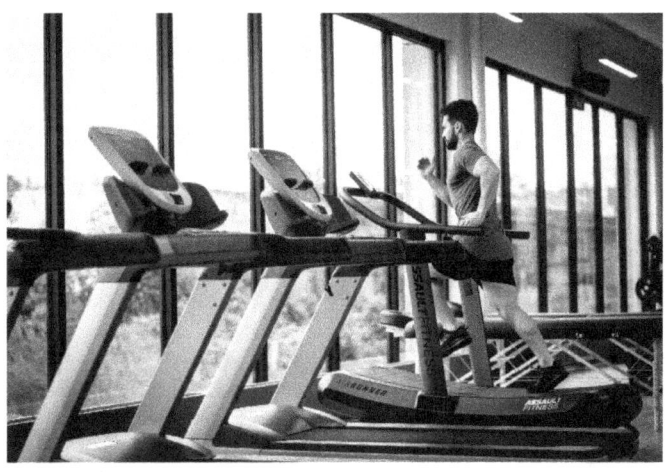

**Thank you for reading please kindly drop your
comments and for more books by me kindly visit
my
Author Center page**

Stay safe